Pregnancy Nutrition

Before, During, & After Eating Tips

By Cathy Wilson

Copyright © 2015

Income Disclaimer

This book contains business strategies, marketing methods and other business advice that, regardless of my own results and experience, may not produce the same results (or any results) for you. I make absolutely no guarantee, expressed or implied, that by following the advice below you will make any money or improve current profits, as there are several factors and variables that come into play regarding any given business.

Primarily, results will depend on the nature of the product or business model, the conditions of the marketplace, the experience of the individual, and situations and elements that are beyond your control.

As with any business endeavor, you assume all risk related to investment and money based on your own discretion and at your own potential expense.

Liability Disclaimer

By reading this book, you assume all risks associated with using the advice given below, with a full understanding that you, solely, are responsible for anything that may occur as a result of putting this information into action in any way, and regardless of your interpretation of the advice.

You further agree that our company cannot be held responsible in any way for the success or failure of your business as a result of the information presented in this book. It is your responsibility to conduct your own due diligence regarding the safe and successful operation of your business if you intend to apply any of our information in any way to your business operations.

Terms of Use

You are given a non-transferable, "personal use" license to this book. You cannot distribute it or share it with other individuals.

Also, there are no resale rights or private label rights granted when purchasing this book. In other words, it's for your own personal use only.

I'm not Perfect...But I'm REAL

Please understand I can't yet afford a fancy-dancy publishing company to present my passionately written books perfectly - Not yet anyway! :)

TRANSLATION - Please don't blast me about the odd spelling error missed. Focus on what you gain.

My Knowledge is For You

Perfect to me is when my fingers take over and dance across the keys. And if you gain just one piece of useful information from my creation, then I'm smiling!

Lastly, without reviews my books will not rank and they will not sell. That's important to me. I have 6 kids to feed! LOL- So, if you've a minute to spare and enjoyed my masterpiece, I'll be tickled rainbow if you left me a review. I'll even owe you one if you like!

Thanks for your time. Enjoy the show!

Cathy :)

Pregnancy Nutrition

Before, During, & After Eating Tips

By Cathy Wilson

Table of Contents

Introduction 11

Chapter One - Why Your Growing Body Needs
Optimal Nutrition in a Nutshell 13

Chapter Two - Key Nutrients You and Your Growing
Baby Need 17

Chapter Three - Important Foods to Eat.................23

Chapter Four - Foods to Avoid..............................29

Chapter Five - Tips to Eating While Preparing For
Pregnancy 35

Chapter Six - Tips For Healthy Eating During
Pregnancy 39

Chapter Seven - Tips for Restorative Eating After
Delivery..47

Chapter Eight - Sample Pregnancy Menu 57

Final Thoughts 61

Introduction

I am not perfect...But I am REAL

Pregnancy Nutrition: Before, During, and After Eating Tips is an introductory guide offering expert nutrition advice to get your body and mind set for a successful pregnancy. You'll learn simple take-action pointers to help nourish your growing baby, deter preventable disease and conditions, serve up the energy required to sail positively through pregnancy, get your body back faster, and fill lost body stores of vitamins, minerals, and other depleted essential nutrients after the birth.

Pregnancy serves up gynormous physical and mental demands on your body. And because you've got a little being dependent on you for food, you need the knowledge to ensure you're making the best choices you can for you and your precious baby.

This is your best place to start to learn better pregnancy nutrition!

Chapter One - Why Your Growing Body Needs Optimal Nutrition in a Nutshell

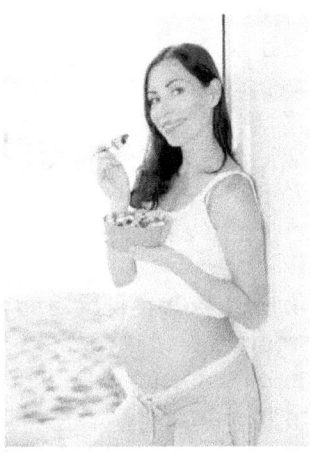

According to *American Pregnancy*, one of the greatest gifts you can give your unborn child is nutritious eating. How you eat before, during, and after pregnancy determines the health of you and your baby. For instance, serious issues like pre-term delivery, autism, and brain development complications increase if adequate iron isn't available throughout pregnancy, according to hemotology.org.

FACT: It's never too late to start eating nutritious food for your growing baby!

Healthy eating before and during pregnancy will...

*Increase fertility
*Prevent minor pregnancy issues
*Increase energy and support positive attitude
*Establish the essential building blocks for optimal growth
*Speed up the recover process after delivery
*Help control weight gain
*Flip your switch to positive throughout pregnancy

Food affects you mentally and physically. What you eat determines how your body works, what you look and feel like, how
you grow and heal, and how much energy is available and uti-
lized now and throughout life.

Your unborn baby depends on you to provide the macronutri-
ents, and essential vitamins and minerals necessary for a
healthy life start, and positive future.

CIP - Cathy's Important Point - The *American Dietician As-
sociation* states incorporating wholesome veggies, lean meats,
fruits, whole grains and legumes, and other wise-owl foods
choices into your daily eating before, during, and after pregnancy, ensures a strong healthy start for your little one. And
with this a faster recovery for mom!

Throughout pregnancy your body cells are busy dividing. Everything from blood volume, nails, hair, breasts, uterus and your
cervix are growing like mad.

Note - American pregnancy experts report your uterus is about
the size of an orange before pregnancy. By the time you're
ready to give birth it's about the size of a watermelon. That's
freakin crazy!

All this growing requires energy. Your hormones are shooting
through the roof, and estrogen and progesterone are the chief
pregnancy hormones.

Healthline reports, when you're pregnant you'll produce more estrogen in one pregnancy, than in your whole life when you're not pregnant!

Estrogen is essential for the optimal growth and supportive function of your placenta throughout pregnancy. This hormone also encourages fetal growth and development, triggers nausea early in pregnancy, is a major player in milk duct development in the second trimester, and peaks somewhere in the third trimester.

Your baby develops and grows at an incredible rate. At just 2 months, your baby is about the size of a kidney bean, moving constantly, with developed webbed fingers.

In just one more month, at 3 months, your baby is about 3 inches long, and already has unique fingerprints.

At 5 months, your baby measures in at about 11 inches long, and has eyelids and eyebrows. And at 8 months of age, your unborn baby has well developed lungs, is putting on layers of fat, and weighs just under 5 pounds.

In order for all of this miraculous growth to happen, you've gotta provide adequate nutrition to ensure optimization of all growth dynamics. A healthy baby is dependent on mom supplying a wide range of healthy food throughout pregnancy.

Small meals throughout the day are also recommended to help keep energy level, deter blood glucose from spiking, and to ensure moods stabilize. And particularly if you're battling nausea, gynormous meals are something you're smart to steer clear of.

Recommendation - *WebMd* recommends all expecting moms take a prenatal vitamin before, during, and after pregnancy. This helps make sure you're providing the best chance for your baby to get a healthy happy start in life!

TIDBIT TIP - I found a prenatal supplement was hard on my stomach, particularly in the first 6 weeks. It helped to have my vitamin with some whole grain toast or a banana.

My Thoughts...

You are what you eat. The birth process is simple amazing. Intricately detailed processes that combine to form all the major components of your baby. Essential organs, blood, vessels and veins, bones, cartilage, tissue, ears, hair, nails, finger and toes. Your baby's entire being is directly influenced and dependent on the healthy nourishment it receives from you.

And we're talking more than healthy eating. Your attitude and mental health. Natural Baby Pros say a mom's emotions affect her unborn child. Experts agree positive thinking can shape the body, help it heal internally, and support healthy growth of your baby during pregnancy.

Eating a balanced nourishing diet will reflect your mental well-being.

Chapter Two - Key Nutrients You and Your Growing Baby Need

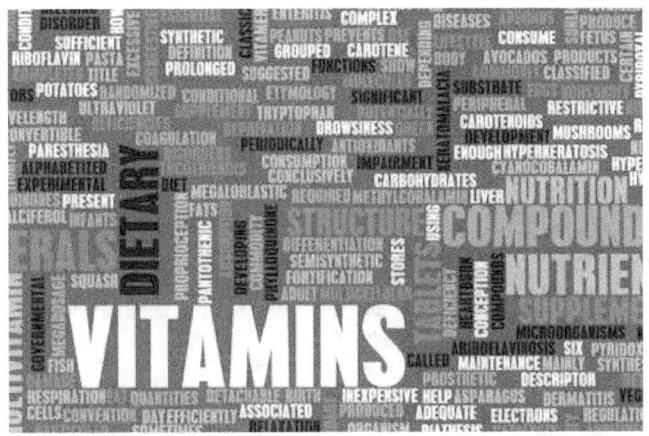

There are lots of different vitamins and minerals your growing baby needs to support optimal health. A key rule of thumb is to eat a diverse range of fresh veggies and fruits, lean protein sources, and healthy complex carbohydrates, like whole grains. And don't forget about getting your protective omega fatty acids at least twice a week. Fatty fish like tuna and salmon are excellent sources.

Take Note - Prenatal vitamins offer many of these nutrients. However natural sources are always your best route.

Nutrients for Optimal Baby Growth

Calcium

Benefits - Muscle development, strong bones and teeth, strong heart, healthy nerve function, supports smooth heart function, and encourages blood clotting.

Daily Requirement - 1000-1200 mg

Sources - 2x2 inch cube cheese (220 mg), 1/2 cup yogurt (250 mg), 1/2 cup cottage cheese (220 mg), 1 cup milk (300 mg), 3/4 cup calcium-fortified vitamin D (250 mg)

FOLIC ACID

Benefits - Helps reduce the risk of developing neural tube defects; essential for healthy gene production; and decreases the risk of other serious birth defects.

Daily Requirement - Approximately 600 mcg

Sources - 1/2 cup soybeans (250 mcg), 1/2 cup spinach (130 mcg), 1/2 cup broccoli (100 mcg), 1/2 avocado (80 mcg), 1/2 cup whole grain pasta (140 mcg)

Copper

Benefits - Ensures proper development and function of blood vessels, nervous system, arteries, heart, and other internal circuitry.

Daily Requirement - About 1 mg

Sources - 1/4 cup cashews (.6 mg), 3 ounces crab meat (1 mg), 3/4 cup kidney beans (.4 mg)

Choline

Benefits - Supports nervous system development, including the brain and neural tube.

Daily Requirement - About 450 mg

Sources - Hard-boiled egg (110 mg), 3-4 ounces white fish (75 mg), 3-4 ounces pork (80 mg)

Vitamin C

Benefits - Important for tissue repair and the creation of collagen, necessary for maintenance of skin, bones, and cartilage.

Daily Requirement - Approximately 85 mg

Sources - 3/4 cup broccoli (75 mg), 1 cup orange juice (100 mg), 3/4 cup cantaloupe (40 mg), 3/4 cup strawberries (75 mg)

Vitamin D

Benefits - Supports strong bones and teeth.

Daily Requirement - At least 5 mcg

Sources - 1 cup skim milk (2 mcg), 3-4 ounces wild salmon (10 mcg)

Zinc

Benefits - Necessary for cell growth and genetic production

Daily Requirement - 12 mg

Sources - 3/4 cup firm tofu (3 mg), 3-4 ounces crab (7 mg), 3/4 cup low-fat yogurt (1.5 mg)

Iron

Benefits - Assists in red blood cell production, gives oxygen to cells for growth and function, and supports bone growth, cartilage, and other connective tissue processes.

Daily Requirement - 30 mg - Which is DOUBLE what a non-pregnant woman needs!

Sources - 3-4 ounces lean ground beef (4 mg), 1 cup spinach (7 mg), 1/2 iron-fortified cereal (15 mg), 3/4 cup lentils (5 mg)

Protein

Benefits - Provides energy for muscle maintenance and production, amino acids essential building blocks for life, and supports healthy cells.

Daily Requirement - About 75 grams

Sources - 3-4 ounces poultry (45 grams), 3-4 ounces lean beef (55 grams), 3-4 ounces tuna (30 grams), 1/4 cup nuts (30 grams), egg (5 grams), 1 cup dairy (15 grams), 1 cup legumes (30 grams)

Fiber

Benefits - Helps naturally move toxins out of your body, aids with digestion and deters constipation.

Daily Requirement - About 30 grams

Sources - 1 cup raspberries (8 grams), apples (4.5 grams), 3/4 cup whole grain pasta (5 grams), 3/4 cup oatmeal (3 grams), 3/4 cup lentils (12 grams), 3/4 cup broccoli (4 grams), 3/4 cup green peas (6 grams)

Omega - 3 Fatty Acids (DHA/EPA)

Benefits - Critical for brain health (DHA) and cell structure (EPA).

Daily Requirement - About 1,000 mg

Sources - 3-4 ounces salmon (1100 mg), 1 enriched egg (250 mg), 3 ounces sardines (2,000 mg), 3-4 ounces mussels (750 mg)

Other Nutrients Essential to Healthy Baby and Mom Are...

Phosphorus

Pantothenic Acid

Riboflavin

Potassium

Vitamin A

Magnesium

Riboflavin

Thiamine

Chromium

Iodine

Manganese

Note - By eating a healthy balanced diet with plenty of fresh veggies, fruits, energy sustaining complex carbohydrates, lean protein, and those essential omega fatty acids, you will provide all the essential vitamins and minerals your body needs throughout pregnancy.

My Thoughts...

Healthy nutrition is a balancing act. And it's important you pay close attention to the foods you're eating when you're expecting, because your little one depends on YOU. Take note most healthcare providers recommend a pre-natal multivitamin before, during, and even after pregnancy, particularly when breastfeeding. This just makes sure you're providing optimal nutrients for your baby's growth, even on the odd occasion you can't provide it.

Use this information to get you started on the right foot for providing your baby with the best nutritional beginning possible!

Chapter Three - Important Foods to Eat

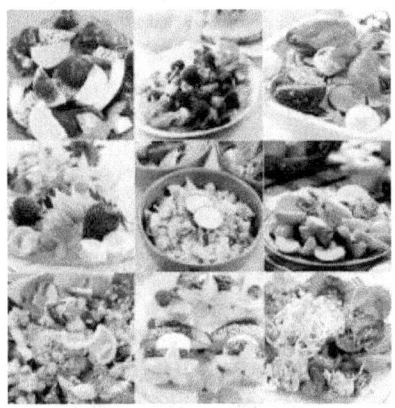

Now we're going to have a look at the actual foods you should be incorporating into your daily diet throughout pregnancy. Keep in mind many of these foods provide nutrients that can't be stored or manufactured by the body, like protein. So you need to ensure you get adequate amounts EVERY day. Protein is required in order for your body to absorb fat-soluble vitamins for one, and to build strong lean muscle.

Protein

How Come: They're the building blocks of life. Every cell in your body and the body of your growing baby has and requires protein for optimal development and function.

How Much: The *American Nutrition Guide* recommends 2-3 servings each day of lean protein.

Serving Size: One small 3-4 ounce chicken breast, a piece of beef about the size of a deck of cards, 1 egg, 3/4 cup legumes, 1/2 cup quinoa, 1 cup milk, 3/4 cup yogurt, 3/4 cup cottage cheese, 1-2 tbsp. peanut butter, 1/4 cup nuts, 2x2 inch cube of real cheese

Protein Foods: Beef, chicken, turkey, ham, eggs, quinoa, milk products, hard cheese, legumes, peanut butter, nuts, and seeds

Protein Deficiency Can Cause: Protein deficiency in mom can cause unexplained weight loss, extreme fatigue, lots of infections, and extreme fluid retention or swelling. *Livestrong* reports lack of protein can trigger abnormal cell growth for your baby. In the final trimester if your baby doesn't get enough protein, mental function issues may develop.

Carbohydrates

How Come: Healthy complex carbs are essential for long-term energy and fiber, which helps to clear waste out of your body. Good carb food sources also contain phytonutrients that act as antioxidants. Think of them as a means of fighting of nasty disease triggering free radicals. These nutrients offer protection for your baby and strengthened immune system function.

CIP - Cathy's Important Point - There's a gynormous difference between simple (bad) carbs and complex (good) carbs.

Simple carbs send blood glucose levels through the roof, provide short-lived energy, and are a direct trigger of diabetes, according to *Medline Today*. Bad carbs are found in high-calorie fast foods and sweets in particular. Donuts, pastries, cakes, cookies, juice, muffins, candy, numerous condiments, and processed foods are the culprits.

FACT - Fruits are simple sugar foods but these are natural sugars that come with added nutrient value.

How Much: Approximately 6-8 servings per day is what's recommended throughout pregnancy.

Serving Size: 3/4 cup whole grain pasta or rice, 6-8 whole grain crackers, 1 piece of fruit, 3/4 cup fruit cup, 1 slice whole wheat bread, 1/3 cup cooked steel cut oats, 1/2 bagel, 1 small sweet potato, 3/4 peas or other veggies

Carbohydrate Foods: Whole grain cereal, bread, pasta, rice, tortillas, pitas, veggies, fruits, sweet potato, bagel

NOTE - You don't get carbohydrates from meat!

Carbohydrate Deficiency Can Cause: Seriously low birth weight. This can also increase the levels of toxic chemicals or ketones in your blood, according to *Baby Center*. Ketones are the waste produced when you're burning fat as fuel. Diets like the Atkins and South Beach Diet are examples of sensationalized low-carb diets to the extreme.

Low-carb consequences directly to mom may include extreme tiredness, bad breath, and increased risk of kidney stones.

Fat

How Come: Fats are essential forms of energy, and help metabolize vitamins A, D, E, and K.

There's a difference in the types if fats your growing body requires. For simplicity, we're going to put fats into 2 categories; good (unsaturated fat) and bad (saturated fat).

Unsaturated Fat - These are the healthy fats your body needs. They are usually liquid at room temperature.

Saturated Fat - These unhealthy fats are solid at room temperature and are typically found in fast foods, sweet treats, and processed "fake" foods. Butter, lard, and palm oil are typical examples of these artery clogging fats.

Trans fats are the most deadly of the bunch. This is synthetic fat that's produced at a low cost and offers a longer shelf life, better aesthetic food appeal, more stable molecules, and enhanced color and flavor. Just think deep fried burgers and fries, pop tarts, TV dinners, and packaged muffins.

Keep in mind that a teeny tiny amount of saturated trans fat is naturally found in animal products like meat, cheese and yogurt. But according to *Mayo Clinic*, studies show minimal amounts of these fats have protective qualities, like reducing the risk of certain cancers.

Natural is always your better choice!

How much: 2-3 servings per day is plenty.

Serving Size: 1-2 tablespoons oil or salad dressing, 1-2 tablespoons nut butter, 1/4 avocado, 3-4 olives, 1 tablespoon mayo, 1/4 cup nuts

Fat Foods (Healthy): Fatty fish like salmon, olive oil, sesame oil, almond oil, corn oil, avocado, olives, peanut butter, nuts and seeds

Fat Deficiency Can Cause: For mom she'll be hungry all the time, skin will get dry, trouble keeping warm, neurological issues like concentrating, and no monthly period. If you aren't getting enough fat to support a pregnancy, your body will stop ovulating and you won't be able to get pregnant. Nature's way of forcing you to get healthy.

Your growing baby may end up born pre-mature with low birth weight, or have issues with brain and eye development if enough healthy fat isn't provided throughout pregnancy.

Pregnancy in NOT the time to diet!

Water

How Come: Water transports vital nutrients and oxygen throughout your body. Without it your body couldn't function and you wouldn't be reading my fantabulous beginner pregnancy book!

Water also helps ensure electrolyte balance, which is key to smooth internal circuitry function. It helps with digestion, transporting waste out of your body, providing energy, regulating internal body temperature, lubricating body parts, and helping with electrical messages that enable your body to move.

How much: dummies.com recommends at least 6-8 glasses per day. If you're exercising regularly, live in a humid climate, or have health issues, you may want to up it a few notches.

Rule of Thumb...Carry a water bottle with you and make a habit of sipping it throughout the day.

Dehydration Can Cause: According to *Medical News Today*, dehydration (from the Greek word *hydro* (water) and the Latin prefix *de-* (which means separation), happens when more water leaves your body than enters.

75% of your body is made of water.

Dehydration may cause thirst, no sweat, dark sunken eyes, confusion, weakness, loss of coordination, dry skin, low blood pressure, heart palpitations, increased temperature, and fainting.

For the baby this causes undo stress. It can deprive the baby of essential nutrients for optimal growth, trigger pre-term deliver, and/or cause retarded in-utero growth.

PREVENTION is critical. Make sure you have 6-8glasses of water each day. And if you suffer from severe morning sickness and are unable to keep hydrated, head straight to Emergency to get the proper medical care.

Other "water" sources - Clear soups and teas are also consider healthy alternative to water. You want to steer clear of soda, energy drinks, juice, and fancy coffee for the most part. These beverages just add oodles of sugar and fatty calories your body doesn't need, with zero nutritional value.

My Thoughts...

It's important to know what types of food and in what amount you should be eating when you're expecting. Your health and the health of your unborn baby are the most important factors bar none.

If you want to think of it in a plate format, you'll want half your plate filled with fresh veggies and some fruit, two-thirds of what's left should be complex carbs like whole grain breads and pasta, beans, and the final third lean protein, eggs, milk product, and lean meat food choices.

Now that you've got a solid understanding of what you should be eating for you and your baby, let's take a peek at what to avoid.

Chapter Four - Foods to Avoid

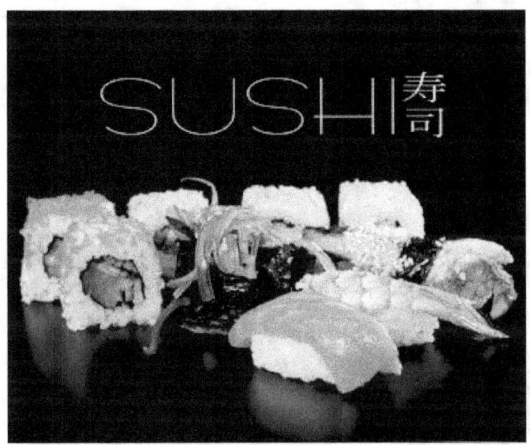

Foodsafety.gov says that because pregnancy affects your immune system function. Both you and your baby are at an increased risk for viruses, parasites, and disease in general. And just because you don't feel "sick," doesn't mean your unborn baby isn't battling off bugs like Listeria. Which may cause serious health complications with your baby.

Make sure all meats are well cooked, and steer clear of...

Soft Cheeses (Brie, Cambembert, queso blanco)

Why... They may have Listeria or E. coli

Safe Option... Go for hard cheese like Swiss or cheddar

Raw Fish - Sushi

*Why...*Could have bacteria or parasites

*Safe Option...*Make sure fish is well cooked

Unpasteurized Milk

*Why...*High risk of containing Salmonella, Listeria, E.coli, or other bacteria

*Safe Option...*Opt for pasteurized milk

Quirky Note - *It's important to note that your individual up-bringing influences your tolerances for certain foods. Nothing is written in concrete. I grew up on a farm and from the time I was 9 months old until I left for university at age 18, I drank unpasteurized cow milk straight from the milk tank. My mom also drank it throughout all of her 5 pregnancies.*

Funny how we all have incredibly strong immune systems, rarely get sick, don't have any serious health issues, maintain healthy weights by eating REAL food, and are generally happy, successful people.

There seem to be too many "rules" today and "fake" foods, that interfere with building strong immune systems and function. Forcing you to learn to sift through all the crap to find the best of the worst, if that makes sense!

Pre-Made Salads Left Out

*Why...*Salads left out at room temperature are fantabulous breeding grounds for bacteria. Ham salad, seafood salad, and egg salad are particularly nasty, according to *WebMD*. FRESH is the name of the game.

Safe Option...Make your salads at home. Ensure everything is fresh. And when you prep meat make sure it's cooked thoroughly and cut on a separate meat cutting board to be safe.

Alfalfa/Bean Sprouts

Why...Breeding grounds for Salmonella and E. coli

Safe Option...Cook them or skip them

BE CAUTIOUS OF...

Deli Meats/Hot Dogs/Sausages

Why...Could be harboring Listeria

Safe Option...Look to eat well done free-range natural meats that are lower fat (chicken, turkey, pork tenderloin)

Undercooked Eggs

Why...May be carrying Salmonella

Safer Option...Make sure anything you eat with eggs is cooked thoroughly

Chicken or Turkey Stuffing

Why...If meat is undercooked it may contain bacteria

Safer Option...Cook stuffing separately to be safe

My Thoughts...

Just use common sense here. Remember these are all just precautions for worst-case scenarios. Don't eat raw chicken, creamy salads that have been on the counter all afternoon, or anything else you aren't normally used to eating.

Don't too excited if you happen to unknowingly eat some un-pasteurized soft cheese, or anything else for that matter. Just relax, eat healthy and smart, and steer around these controversial foods if you can.

LISTERIA FEATURE (Listeria is rare)

What is Listeria?

It's a bacteria found in soil and water. Animals can carry it along with veggies, cuz they come from the earth. Unpasteurized milk can also carry, including foods made from it.

VIP - You can kill Listeria by cooking food!

What are the Risks of Getting Listeria When Pregnant?

CDC (Center of Disease Control) estimates just 1700 people in the US get seriously ill from Listeria each year. Even though pregnant women are 20 times more likely to develop this disease than non-pregnant women, just 17% of these cases involve pregnant women.

Symptoms...

Symptoms may show up immediately, or up to a month later. They range from flu symptoms, fever, muscle aches, and vomiting, to more severe symptoms including, stiff neck, confusion, and convulsions.

When this disease sneaks into the nervous system it becomes red alert serious.

Note - According to experts at *American Pregnancy*, your greatest time to develop Listeria is in your final trimester, when your immune system function is the weakest.

Will Listeria Harm My Baby?

If you're pregnant with Listeria the risk increases for...

*Miscarriage
*Pre-term deliver
*Newborn with infection
*Newborn death (stillbirth or death shortly after)

Treatment Options

Most cases are successfully treated with antibiotics. This usually protect the baby from developing Listeria. Newborns with Listeria will also be administered antibiotics.

Prevention Moves

*Wash and cook all food thoroughly
*Eat hard cheese
*Stay away from processed deli meat
*Don't eat fish unless it's fresh and cooked well

Chapter Five - Tips to Eating While Preparing For Pregnancy

Pre-conception nutrition is essential to a healthy pregnancy. What you eat when preparing your body for pregnancy is directly responsible for your health throughout pregnancy and the health of your developing fetus.

*If you are overweight, your doctor will advise you to keep your weight gain on the lower end because you've an increased risk of pregnancy issues arising like elevated blood pressure or gestational diabetes.

*Underweight women may need to put on a little extra weight to avoid a small birth weight baby.

*Experts at *URMC Health* state for normal weight women, 20-30 pounds in suggested. Speak with your healthcare provider to help you figure out you best weight gain plan.

MyPlateGov simplifies the big picture by mentioning the focus should be on eating a balanced nutritional "big picture"diet.

***Grains** - These include rice, oats, barley, wheat, whole wheat, brown rice, oatmeal, and other grain products.

***Lean Protein** - Pick low-fat meat and poultry, fish, nuts, beans, and seeds.

***Veggies** - Eat a diverse range of veggies. Make sure you include dark leafy greens, and brightly colored veggies like yellow and red peppers, along with legumes and potatoes.

***Dairy Products** - Choose from low-fat milk, yogurt, cottage cheese, pudding, hard cheese, and other low-fat dairy foods.

***Fruits** - All fruits are good to eat. They can be fresh, frozen, canned, diced, sliced, dried, or pureed. Fresher is better, and if you're choosing canned watch for added sugar.

***Animal Fats** - You should steer clear of these.

***Healthy Oils** - In moderation oils like peanut oil, olive oil, and corn oil are important in optimal health.

**Folic Acid Note* - Nutrition experts recommend .4 mg of folic acid daily for women of childbearing years. Found in leafy greens, oranges, beans, nuts and seeds, and fortified whole grain breakfast cereals.

This will help ensure your baby's spinal cord fuses shut properly, avoiding paralysis, incontinence, or mental disability.

Most neural tube defects occur in the first 28 days after conception, which is often before pregnancy is detected.

Taking a prenatal supplement helps with prevention.

Iron Note - Many young women battle low iron stores because of a diet low in iron and menstruation. By building up your iron stores before conception, you're going to ensure the best environment for your baby to grow.

Key iron sources include:

*Kale, collards, and turnip
*Dark poultry in particular
*Organ meats, beef, and ham
*Oysters and anchovies
*Whole grain pasta, rice, cereal, and bread

BONUS PRE-PREGNANCY TIPS

*See your doctor
*Stop drinking, smoking, and taking recreational drugs (get professional help if required)
*Take pre-natal vitamin
*Ditch the processed fast food and opt for clean eating
*Limit caffeine intake to 1-2 cups daily or less
*Find your healthy weight
*Ensure you're exercising at least 3 days/week (30 min. cardio, 15 minutes weights)
*Have dental checkup
*Get finances in order
*Ensure your mental health is good
*Take up yoga or meditate
*Figure out when you ovulate
*Make sure your environment is healthy

The guys often get the short end of the stick here. Plannedparenthood.org says the fathers-to-be need to buckle down and follow suit with the mom-to-be. This includes getting a checkup to make sure everything's in order, eating healthier, exercising regularly, and reducing stress.

Here are a few habits that affect sperm count negatively...

*Smoking
*Drinking
*Drugs
*Steroids
*Heated tubs, saunas, or whirlpools
*Some over-the-counter medicine and prescription drugs

My Thoughts...

Having a new baby is a big deal. And taking the time to prepare as much as possible is a wise-owl move on your part. Whether you're pregnant or not, it's important to take care of you. When you're looking at the possibility of having a baby, the stakes just rose up a few levels.

Talk with your doctor or nutrition expert about getting set with healthy eating and lifestyle moves BEFORE the stick turns pink or blue.

Chapter Six - Tips For Healthy Eating During Pregnancy

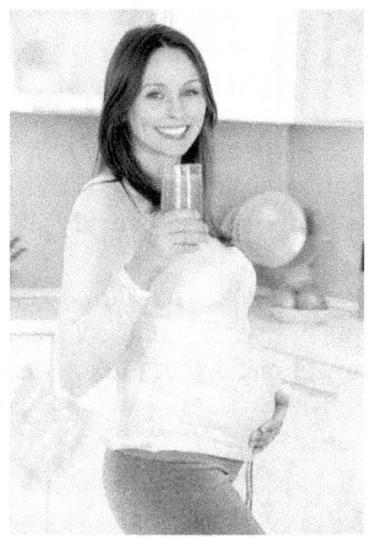

I need you to remove the thought from your brain right now that you're eating for two when pregnant. That's just an excuse to get fat and unhealthy. The growing baby you're supporting for 9 months requires very little extra energy. In fact, *Healthy Living* experts state you need just 300 extra calories daily in the last trimester to support baby growth.

To get that into perspective for you, that's a...

Whole grain bagel with cream cheese
Or
Banana, 1 cup skim milk, 1 hard-boiled egg
Or

1/2 cup mixed nuts
Or
1 cup cooked oatmeal with milk, 1cup mixed fruit
Or
3/4 cup whole grain pasta with tomato sauce, 1 small grilled chicken breast

That's it!

Not much is it?

Here are a few healthy eating tips to set you up for a smooth pregnancy and quick delivery!

*NEVER Skip Breakfast - If your tummy is upset, try some whole grain crackers or dry toast. Otherwise, maybe opt for healthy dish of oatmeal made with milk and a banana, or perhaps a poached egg with wheat bread and a glass of fresh squeezed orange juice.

Just get something in your tummy!

*Have Healthy Snacks in Reach - Make sure you've got fresh fruit, veggies, nuts and seeds, yogurt, real cheese, peanut butter, whole grain bread, and other healthy snacks in reach when hunger strikes. This isn't the time to fill up on processed fast food junk.

*Up the Water and the Fiber - Fibrous foods like beans, fresh fruits and veggies, whole grains and brown rice, are going to give you the fiber required to keep things moving along nicely. Adding 6-8 glasses of water per day to this will give your body the means of purging harmful toxins, while keeping constipation far, far away.

*Be Certain to Get Your Folic Acid and Iron Daily - Taking a pre-natal supplement makes certain you get the iron and folic acid your developing baby needs for optimal health. Iron will help to keep your blood flowing healthy, and folic acid's going to deter serious birth defects.

*Get 2-3 Servings Per Week Fish - *Medicinenet* recommends salmon, shrimp and shellfish. Just be sure to steer clear of high mercury fish like shark and swordfish.

*Pay Attention to Your Hunger - It's natural to have a poor appetite the first few months when the nausea often strikes. Small bland snacks often seem to work best while your body if adjusting to pregnancy. Throughout the middle of your pregnancy your hunger will likely be similar to your usual appetite when not pregnant. It's the final three months where you're likely to kick into high gear with eating. It's also more uncomfortable to eat more because your stomach's getting squished and heartburn is often more prevalent. This is a good time to flip back to mini-meals often, so you don't end up feeling icky constantly.

Listen to your hunger cues and you're doing the right thing.

*Talk With Your Doctor About Food Restrictions - For personal reasons, like vegan or religious beliefs, you may need professional guidance to ensure you're getting all the essential vitamins and minerals your body needs to support baby growth.

*Watch How You Cook Your Food - Cooking the crap out of your veggies, or dropping a healthy chicken breast into the deep fryer, takes a good thing and kills it. The overcooking steals vital nutrients, and the deep frying adds oodles of unwanted fat and calories to your meal. None of which are good for you or your growing baby.

Cooking options should be...

*Baking
*Broiling
*Steaming
*Poaching
*Barbecuing
*Grilling

Steer Clear of the Extras - You don't need to add oodles of fattening sour cream and butter to your baked potato. When cooking you can use cooking spray, or drizzle olive oil in pan and wipe out the excess. Put a touch of mustard or barbecue sauce on your sandwich instead of mayo or creamy sauces. And drizzle low-fat salad dressing on your leafy greens instead of making a swimming pool with it.

Easy on the condiments to help control excess fat and sugar.

Naked eating rocks!
Choose Low-Fat Dairy Products - You don't need homo milk and full fat yogurt when pregnant. Look for low-fat varieties to help keep your fat intake down. Many milk products are loaded with fat, and you don't need it!

MODERATION is the key.

Have a Target Weight - It's critical to not use pregnancy as reason to throw panties to the wind, eating as much as you want of everything. Guidelines vary, and according to **parents.com**, the rough guidelines for weight gain are...

-20 to 35 pounds when normal weight to start
-25-40 pounds when underweight
-15-25 pounds when overweight
-35-45 pounds with twins

Now's Not the Time to Diet - If you're overweight and pregnant, and find you're pushing the scale up too quickly, don't diet, just make some healthier eating adjustments. Drink non-fat milk instead of 2%, and go for low-fat yogurt instead of the full-fat version. Choose fresh fruits instead of high sugar snacks. Lean meats instead of fattier cuts are a smart move. And toss out the sugary fruit juices and soda for good old-fashioned water.

Stop and think about what you're eating cuz there's always room for improvement!

*Protein - Your body needs about 10 extra grams of protein each day to support fetal growth. You don't get this from your pre-natal vitamin, so ensure you're eating 2-3 servings each day of protein-rich foods.

Protein-Rich Foods - Low-fat dairy products, lean beef, soy, eggs, lentils, beans, spinach, nuts and seeds, chicken, turkey, and nut butters.

*Don't Skimp on Calcium - It helps support bone growth, healthy gums, teeth, and hair. Mom also needs it to prevent osteoporosis down the road.

Great Calcium Foods - Orange juice that's calcium fortified, hard cheese, milk, yogurt, pudding, cottage cheese, almonds, seaweed, and broccoli.

*Same As Pre-Pregnancy Suggestions With Fiber - Even more so, you want to ensure you're getting adequate fiber to help you feel full, and deter hemorrhoids and constipation.

Smart Fiber Foods - Whole grain pasta, rice, breads and cereals, apples and pears with skin, berries, oranges, veggies, nuts and seeds.

*Get Your Healthy Fat in Moderation - You know fat helps develop your baby's brain and central nervous system, while transporting nutrients and acting as energy.

By eating 2-3 servings per day of healthy fat foods, you're getting plenty.

*Healthy Fat Options - 1/4 avocado, 3-4 olives, 1-2 tablespoons olive oil, sunflower oil, corn oil, salmon, and nuts.

HEALTHY SNACK IDEAS TO GET THAT 300 EXTRA CALORIES

*3/4 cup low-fat yogurt with 1/4 cup sunflower seeds and banana
*1/2 whole grain bagel toasted with tablespoon peanut butter and apple
*Grilled chicken breast on pumpernickel bun with veggies and slice Swiss cheese
*1/2 cup mixed nuts and cup fresh fruit
*1 cup broccoli, 1 cup spinach, 1 cup carrots stir-fried in 1/4 cup beef both, with 3-4 ounces lean beef
*1 cup low-fat cottage cheese with 20 grapes and a pear
*1 can tuna mixed with tablespoon low-fat mayo, stuffed in half whole grain pita with veggies
*Chicken spinach salad - 2 cups spinach, 1/2 cup mandarin oranges, 1/4 cup sliced almonds, 1   egg chopped, and drizzle low-fat salad dressing
*Smoothie - 1/2 cup low-fat yogurt, 1 banana, 1/2 cup blackberries, 1/2 cup raspberries, 1/2 cup blueberries, 1/4 cup skim milk

My Thoughts...

Eating when you're expecting a baby doesn't have to be complicated. And if you have questions, make sure you speak to your healthcare provider or doctor. In a nutshell, you want to get 2-3 servings each day of lean protein, plenty of healthy carbs in fruits, veggies and beans, fiber from your fruits and veggies, calcium from dairy products, spinach and broccoli, omega fatty acids from fresh fish, salmon in particular, lots of water, and of course moderate amounts of healthy fats.

By eating a healthy diverse range of natural unprocessed foods, you'll have no issues providing essential nutrients for your baby and body, while keeping your weight in check!

Chapter Seven - Tips for Restorative Eating After Delivery

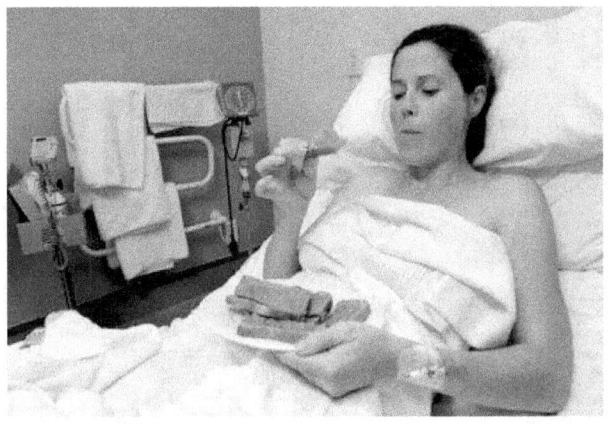

Now that the main event is over, and your beautiful new baby is born, it's more important to provide your body with optimal nutrition. If you're breast feeding, your baby is still 100% dependent on you for fuel. It's also critical to eat well to refill lost energy stores, and keep your energy up in your day to day. Particularly when you're often running on little to no sleep in the beginning.

Parenting Today, states weight loss is the number one priority, aside from taking care of your baby that women focus on after the birth. This makes perfect sense. Psychologically you've likely had enough. For NINE long months your body was rented out and now that you finally get it back, you want to fix it fast, cuz it's been stretched and bent out of shape, along with lots of fat padding attached.

Just like letting someone borrow your skinny suit and returning fat pants that really don't fit, at least in your mind.

Pointers to Get Your Body Back Fast Through Nutrition

*Eat to Get Energized! - Sure the sleepless nights are going to whack you pretty hard. But it's the food you put on your plate that also reflects whether or not you've got the energy required to stay awake and feel able to care for your little one.

Eat small amounts of nutritious wholesome foods throughout the day to help deter moods swings, energy cliffs, and that sickly draggy feeling like you're fresh off a hangover. Registered dietician *Kathy McManus*, a board member on the Nutrition Program at Brigham Women's Hospital in Boston, believes mini-meals are essential in maintaining every levels.

*Focus on Getting the Key Nutrients - By eating healthy key nutrients you'll provide the food your growing baby needs, along with helping with the mentality required to handle all the stresses associated with being a new mom.

The basic key nutrients to tune into are:

-Plenty of veggies and fresh fruit
-Healthy whole grains to help sustain energy levels longer and provide ample fiber to push waste away
-Lean meat for fast energy, muscle building, and ensuring your body can absorb all those fat soluble vitamins required by you and your new little one
-Dark leafy greens that offer oodles of vital nutrients, including protective anti-oxidants to help deter disease-creating free radicals from making you sick

-Ensure you're eating plenty of iron-rich foods like spinach, lean meats, and fortified cereals, in order to fight off depression and ensure you've got adequate energy stores to tackle the day
-Vitamin C foods like citrus fruits and tomatoes, will help immensely in the healing process, particularly if you've delivered via C-section

*Have Lots of Small Healthy Snacks on Hand When Hunger Strikes - Experts at *BabyCenter* suggest having healthy snacks prepped and ready to go before you're hungry. Better yet have your partner, friend or family member do the honors while you take a little nap!

Quick Healthy Snack Ideas...

-6 Whole grain pita chips with hummus or light cream cheese
-Homemade nut mixture with raisins and sunflower seeds (1/2 cup)
-3/4 cup low-fat cottage cheese with 10 grapes
-Hard-boiled egg with 2x2 inch cube of cheddar cheese
-3/4 cup yogurt with one sliced banana
-Healthy whole grain granola bar (watch the sugar)
-3/4 cup quinoa with piece of fruit (quinoa one of the few plant based complete protein sources)
-One cup of fresh berries with 1/2 a whole grain bagel and a smear of peanut butter
-Handful of raisins and half a whole wheat pita stuffed with veggies, and 1/2 a grilled chicken breast
-3/4 cup of oatmeal made with skin milk, 1/4 cup slivered almonds, and 1/2 cup blueberries
-3/4 cup whole grain cereal with 1/2 cup skim milk
-Protein smoothie - 1/2 cup low-fat yogurt, 1/2 banana, 1/2 cup mixed berries, scoop protein powder
-Two stalks celery with two tablespoons peanut butter
-Plate with one sliced apple, one sliced pear, ten grapes, and half cup yogurt for dipping
-Egg wrap - whole grain wrap with one egg and veggies

-Peanut butter wrap - whole grain wrap with 1-2 tablespoons peanut butter with lettuce
-Spinach salad - 2 cups fresh spinach, sliced carrots, cucumber and green peppers, sprinkle with sunflower seeds, and drizzle low-fat dressing to taste
-Two cheese strings when you're on the go
-Pudding cup and one banana
-Half a whole grain bagel with 2 tablespoons low-fat cream cheese

*Stay Away From High Sugar Processed Foods - It's too easy to grab a donut, cookies, or some other junky sweet simple sugar treat when you're tired and hungry. Right now your body is recovering from a major transformation. It needs vital minerals and essential nutrients to get healed and strong again. Fast foods and junky sugary sweet treats offer little to no nutritional value, steal energy, are loaded with deadly bad trans fat, have oodles of extra fat calories, and trigger blood sugar spikes that are moving you one step closer to developing diabetes.

Choose to eat natural foods and you'll get your body back FAST!

*Drink Up! - Whether you're breast feeding or not, right now your body needs oodles of water to help level your hormones and internal circuitry, flush toxins and excess salt that causes bloating, transport vital nutrients throughout your body, and to provide essential energy to keep you ticking!

BabyCenter experts agree 6-8 glasses of the crystal clear stuff is you baseline. And when you're breastfeeding, you should have a nice big glass of water of tea to drink before, during, and after every feed. Remaining hydrated is critical to your good health, the health of your baby, and losing the baby fat that's driving your bonkers!

*Up Your Oats! - Eating your oats provides oodles of calcium, iron, good carbs, fiber, and protein. All essential nutrients you need to recover and provide. Adding fresh fruit, in particular berries, will up protective antioxidants. This helps strengthen immune system function, and keep your mind and body strong!

*The Indian Culture Has it Right! - Turmeric is loaded with fiber, potassium, vitamin B6 and C, magnesium, and manganese to start. These essential nutrients are exactly what your body is looking for.

Indians have used turmeric for centuries for healing and wound treatment. So it makes sense this is something that'll help your body recover internally. Using it for cooking is great. Or you can just add about a teaspoon to a glass of milk.

*Almonds - Almonds are rich in complex carbohydrates, E and B vitamins, fiber, calcium, zinc, copper, and other vital nutrients to propel your system back to normal faster. Almonds are great as a snack solo, or you can add them to anything from salads and stir-fries, to yogurt and cereal.

*Dark and Brightly Colored Veggies - Spinach, romaine lettuce, peppers and squash, are just a few veggies loaded with vital nutrients like iron, vitamin C, and antioxidants that will help build your body strong, while providing energy for your day to day function.

*Up Your Fish - *WebMD* states fish is one of the "superfoods" you should be loading up on after delivery, in order to provide your body with DHA, a vital omega-3 fatty acid that helps your baby develop strong brain and central nervous system function. Salmon, sardines, and tuna canned in water are great options.

CIP- Cathy's Important Point-The debate continues as to whether or not breastfeeding helps mom return to her pre-pregnancy weight faster. Most experts do agree that if you choose to eat healthy nutritious foods in the right amounts, while fitting in regular exercise, breastfeeding moms tend to lose weight faster.

**Breastfeeding does burn about 300 extra calories per day according to nutrition experts at *Dietitians of America*. Something to keep in mind.

Get Moving - This isn't an eating tip per say, but if you want to lose weight and keep it off you've gotta get your butt moving to the beat of exercising. I understand you're feeling tired, bloated, fat and cranky after having your baby, but I promise you'll feel better by easing yourself into some fresh air and exercise.

You gotta start somewhere!

According to *Dr. Shane Shaughnessy*, Ontario, Canada, getting your heart rate up with muscle building and cardiovascular exercise will trigger increased metabolism, release endorphins that'll put you in a good mind, and trigger positive energy release.

Regular exercise also helps you...

-burn fat
-build lean muscle to burn fat and calories
-deters depression
-improves sleep quality
-releases stress

Professor of Kinesiology at Michigan State University, *Dr. James Pivarnik,* suggests started with 150 minutes per week. Don't forget that small bouts of 15-20 minutes each adds up.

Understanding time is tough commodity when you've got a newborn.

Strength training can be done using your baby, a laundry detergent container with a handle, or even a few jars of peanut butter. The idea is to figure out what works for you and build off it.

If you've had a C-section, speak with your doctor about what exercises you can do. Where there's a will, there's a way!

*Get Quality Sleep - I know this is a tough one, but getting sleep when you can is a must. This means sleeping when the baby sleep, accepting help from neighbors, friends and family so you can catch a nap, and go to bed early when you can, even if there's a load of laundry to do.

Studies show women tend to hold onto their extra pregnancy weight if they get less than 5 hours sleep per night. They also choose less nutritious foods. When you're tired you trigger cortisol, a stress hormone that may tip off weight gain. Sound sleep enables you to function, make healthier food choices, and take better care of yourself and your baby.

*Don't Starve Yourself - When you deprive yourself of the minimum number of calories your body requires to function, BMR, your body will turtle and start shutting down. Your metabolism will slow, every carrot stick you eat will be stored as fat for use later, energy won't exist, and you'll feel like crap. Your body will actually fight your intended weight loss because it doesn't trust you, because you're not providing it with the basics.

NEWSFLASH - You've got eat to lose weight. Just eat in moderation and healthy!

Your height, weight, sex, and activity level can be used to calculate your BMR, or minimum calories your body needs to maintain your weight. From here you can figure out what amount of ballpark calories you need to lose weight.

BMR calculators are readily available online to get you started. Or you can have your doctor, nutritionist, or trainer help you figure it out! A fantabulous place to start!

*Beans Please! - Legumes are loaded with iron, fiber, and non-animal protein. An excellent breastfeeding food that's easy on the budget too.

*Brown Rice - So many people are afraid of carbs, even complex carbs, cuz they think carbs promote fat. Especially if you're breastfeeding, don't cut back on good carbs like brown rice, cuz this can cause weight loss too fast, which slows milk production. Not to mention the fact you'll feel sluggish all over. Good carbs are essential in moderation for safe healthy weight loss, according to *WebMD* nutrition experts.

*Calcium-Fortified Orange Juice - Particularly when breastfeeding, oranges are a fabulous route to boosting your energy fast. Having a glass each day of calcium-fortified orange juice when you're breastfeeding is a double win for you and your newborn.

*More Eggs Please! - Eggs are easy-peasy. You can have them boiled, poached, scrambled, diced up in a salad, or wrapped up for a quick lunch. Choosing eggs that are DHA-fortified will provide an essential fatty acid for bonus. An excellent complete protein and iron source to work into your day!

*Balance Snacks - Nutritionally balanced snacks promotes weight loss with providing constant energy. Aim to have your snacks between 200-300 calories, with protein, complex carbs, and good fat in each. This provides the rich mix of energy for your body repair and strengthening.

Example Balanced Snacks...

-One slice whole grain bread with one tablespoon peanut butter, and a pear
-One cup low-fat milk with a banana
-Ten carrot sticks dipped in 1/2 cup hummus, and a cup low-fat hot chocolate
-All-natural protein bar (watch the sugar)
-Two whole grain rice cake with tablespoon peanut butter each and sliced banana
-One cup chocolate milk and 1.5 cups fresh fruit
-Grapes and cheese sticks - cut up two portions of 2x2 in cheese cubes, and alternate with 10-15 grapes, makes about four toothpicks full

My Thoughts...

Getting all the essential nutrients your body needs after childbirth is priority one, aside from caring for your baby. Your body needs to rest and heal. This requires a continuous supply of healthy energy, lots of sleep, and regular exercise.

Take what works and apply. And make certain you run everything past your healthcare provider before implementing, just to be safe.

Chapter Eight - Sample Pregnancy Menu

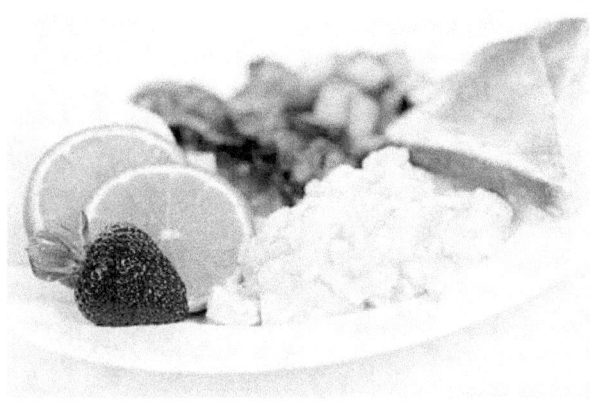

Here's a sample pregnancy menu to give you an idea of what a healthy, balanced, nutritious meal plan looks like to get you started.

Breakfast One

Two slices whole grain toast
Two poached eggs
One cup fresh fruit

Tea/Water

Snack One

One small yogurt
Apple

Banana

Water

Lunch One

Grilled chicken wrap - whole grain tortilla, grilled chicken, veggies
Small whole grain bun
Apple

Water

Snack Two

1/2 cup mixed nuts
Cheese string

Water

Dinner One

Two cups spinach, 3-4 ounces grilled steak, 1/4 cup sunflower seeds, drizzle low-fat dressing
One cup steamed broccoli
One small sweet potato

Water/Tea

Snack Three

One cup cantaloupe
Ten whole grain crackers with smear low-fat cream cheese

Water

Approximate Calories - 2500

Breakfast Two

3/4 cup cooked oatmeal made with low-fat milk
1 cup mixed berries

Tea/Water

Snack Four

One cup veggies sticks with 1/2 cup yogurt dip
3/4 cup pineapple

Water/Tea

Lunch Two

Grilled pork stir-fry - 1 cup sliced pork, 1 cup mixed veggies,
1/4 chicken broth to steam pork and veggies in
Garden salad with drizzles low-fat salad dressing

Water or Tea

Snack Five

3/4 cup low-fat cottage cheese with 1 cup fresh fruit
10 whole grain crackers

Water or tea

Dinner Two

One portion grilled salmon
One cup steamed asparagus
One cup wild rice
One cup diced watermelon, musk melon, pear, apples, and
grapefruit

Water/tea

Snack Six

One banana sliced with two tablespoons nut butter - eat like a
sandwich
Handful roasted almonds

Water/tea

Approximate Calories - 2500

My Thoughts...

*This gives you a base menu to start from. What you're looking
for is to balance each mini-meal or snack with some healthy
lean protein, complex carbs, and good fat. This enables con-
sistent readily available energy throughout the day.*

Hope this helps you get started on the right nutrition track!

Final Thoughts

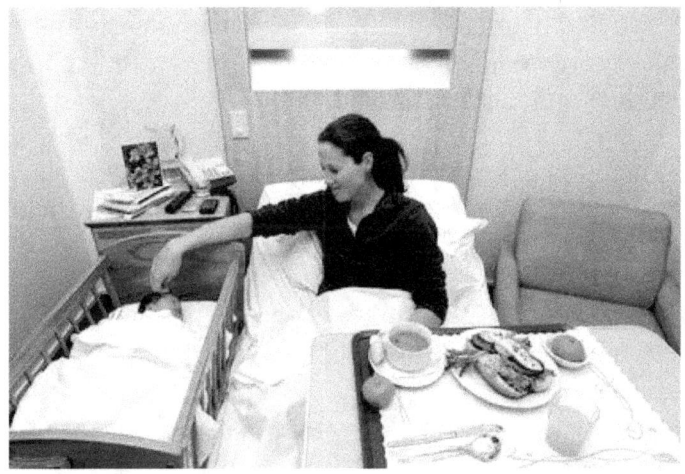

Pregnancy is a special and exciting time in your life. A transition where it's not just about you anymore. Anything and everything you do mentally, physically, nutritionally, environmentally and socially, is now for both your and your baby. A miraculous, but often stressful feeling, a gynormous responsibility.

The *IOM, Institute of Modern Medicine Food and Nutrition Board* and the *American College of Obstetricians and Gynecologists* propose adequate intake of all essential vitamins and minerals for good reason in pregnancy. Countless research studies and findings indicate the health and wellness of the mother before, during, and after delivery, is directly indicative of the overall birthing experience and health of both mother and newborn.

Anything you can learn to *better* your experience should be your natural focus and desire.

All you can do is open your mind to learn about the best food and health choices for *the bigger you*, and apply. It's not about being perfect, cuz nobody is. It's about making better food choices each day to move through pregnancy start to finish with less *preventable* hiccups. So that both you and your baby are healthier and happier throughout.

The sooner you get started the better. And I hope you've gained at least one positive piece of information from this introduction to pregnancy nutrition book. That'll make me one happy camper!

To great health and nutrition, and good luck with your pregnancy!

Cathy :)

Last Thoughts…

*THANK-YOU for reading my masterpiece. I hope you learned a little something, or at least got a fcw smiles.
*I would appreciate a millisecond or three of your time for a quick review, to help me build my masterful book empire higher.
*Whatever you do, don't forget to smile, and of course, check out my website for more of my e-Book masterpieces at: www.flawlesscreativewriting.com

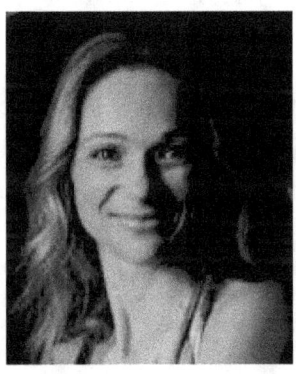

Thank you!
Cathy ☺

Disclaimer

www.ingramcontent.com/pod-product-compliance
Lightning Source LLC
Chambersburg PA
CBHW071118280526
45787CB00003B/1089